Power Plants: Thirty Adaptogens and a Treasure Chest of Useful Herbs

POWER PLANTS, THIRTY ADAPTOGENS AND A TREASURE CHEST OF USEFUL HERBS, FIRST EDITION

Published by johnvajra.com in alliance with Vajra Books.

Printed in the United States of America
First Printing, 2015

ISBN-13: 978-1535326551
ISBN: 978-1535326551

Disclaimer

Power Plants

- Table of Contents -

Calamus
Licorice
Nettles
Gentian
Red Clover
Sarsparilla
Burdock
Angelica
Oatstraw & Oats
Agrimony
True Solomon's Seal
Borage
Calendula
Dandelion
Wild Indigo
Black Cohosh
Fenugreek
Goldenseal
Astragalus
Eleuthero
Rhaponticum
Rhodiola
Turmeric
Ginger
Cinnamon
Brahmi
Holy Basil
Basil
Cayenne
Hawthorn
Rosemary
Pine
Periwinkle
Black Cumin
Cumin
Alfalfa
Thyme

Herb Collections

Herbs for the Mind
Herbs for Headaches

Herbs for Digestion
Herbs for Colds
Herbs for Fever
Herbs for Wounds and Cuts
Herbs for Head Injury
Herbs for Broken Bones
Herbs for Burns and Sunburns
Herbs for Poisonous Bites
Herbs for Bruises Strains and Sprains
Herbs for Boils and Abscesses
Herbs for Tooth Health and Pain
Herbs for Nerve Injuries

Power Plants:
Thirty Adaptogens and a Treasure Chest of Useful Herbs

The world is full of power plants, plants that heal and empower the entire body and its myriad functions. These plants, part of every culture, identified and used over countless generations, and often considered magical and held in extremely high regard, are part of humankind's heritage, and one of the primordial ways of maintaining health, presence and the good functioning of the body.

The concept of an adaptogen herb, in its modern definition, comes from Russia, and was also widely used by Western naturopathic doctors in America until about a century ago. There is a lot of money being made out of the exclusive commercialization of Chinese adaptogen herbs, and quite a bit of suffering resulting from the loss of our own background of natural culture regarding herbs. Much research is being done right now into Western adaptogens, and dozens of plants are coming to light, each with an incredible array of positive, uplifting, life-protective effects. Not all the plants presented here have been officially recognized as adaptogens, but all of them have amazing empowering abilities for a mix of mind and body systems, and can be safely used. These are, each and every one of them, power plants—plants you should build a relationship with and come to know and enjoy fully.

They have allowed men and women to survive and thrive across a large range of conditions in time and space, and they are still around for us to use today. While many of the commonly commercialized adaptogens are used as energy tonics, there is a much wider range of effects and usefulness that needs to be explored, and the plants presented here have deep effects on the heart and mind, on energy systems and the balancing and restorative power of the body. Some are subtly powerful, some are exceedingly so, and all are incredibly useful.

An adaptogen generates direct energy in a way that is full and balanced in body and mind, and works inherently through the cells, organs and systems in an intelligent, continuous, enduring and adaptive manner. It increases the body's inner power and stability while making it perform better against external stressors, and function more positively in the world as a whole. Adaptogens relax mind-body tension, increase resilience to all factors, and replenish lifeforce, energy, and the body's inherent usable power. They are non-toxic and safe to use for long period of time, normalize body functions and the overall defense ability of the body, doing so through many effects, body systems and organs, and despite having a more pronounced action in certain body systems, they restore balance to all systems and the body as a whole. Adaptogens have been widely used in all cultures—the Ayurvedic and Chinese traditions, Native American and African medicine, where they were seen as complex whole body tonics with both wide activity and specific strengths. They were used to resist disease, save the sick from even the most dangerous states of chronic disease and whole body exhaustion, and, in the healthy, to improve all functions, strengthen the lifeforce of tissues, organs and systems, build mind-body energy and balance, and gain full body power, relaxation, vitality and presence.

Remember, this is not medical advice, and you should research any herb you use. Especially if you are pregnant, you should not touch any new subtance before fully researching it.

Disclaimer: The author makes no guarantees regarding the medical or curative effect of any herb or tonic, and no reader should attempt to use any of the information provided here as treatment for any illness, weakness, or disease without first consulting a physician or health care provider. Pregnant women should always consult first with a health care professional before taking any treatment.

Calamus

Calamus was a favorite herb of the Native Indians, who used it as a stimulant, full body tonic, and a powerful adaptogen for the mind and body. In Ayurveda it is seen as a tonic for the brain and one of the best mind herbs, clearing the mental channels and fortifying the mind's ability to obtain information and evoke knowledge from memory, enhancing lifeforce and stimulating the nervous system. It triggers the mind and promotes positive thoughts, empowering focus and concentration, promoting clarity, opening the mind, stabilizing it, organizing speech and correlating attention and thinking. It supports expression and overall nervous health. It has positive effects on learning, recovering from shock, and treating anxiety and depression. It can erase trauma, conquer hysteria, overcome the effects of surgery, stop epilepsy and treat neuralgia. It can even treat mental retardation, over time, and has been shown to help develop speech and expression in children who had never learned to speak. It is a specific for ADD and ADHD, and removes toxic residues and the influence of drugs from the liver, nervous system and brain. Overall, it simply increases intellectual and energetic capacity, clears mental channels and awareness, and allows consciousness to both relax and concentrate directly.

Ancient Egyptians used Calamus root as a powerful aphrodisiac and trusted it with building the health of the reproductive system. All over the world, it was used for restoring health and healing prolonged, chronic sickness, against poison and contagious disease. Native American warriors applied root juices on their faces to drive away fear before battle, and the Turks used it to heal all kinds of infections. Mongol invaders planted Calamus in any water source they wanted to drink from.

Calamus strengthens the digestive system and removes intestinal worms, treats abdominal pain, flatulence, lack of appetite, loss of taste, colds, bronchitis and sinusitis, wounds and inflammation, angina, sore throat, coughs, throat colds, irritable coughs, chest colds, head colds, arthritis, asthma, sinus congestion, headaches, seizures, convulsions, cerebral trauma, amnesia, Alzheimer's, dementia, ulcers and gastritis, diarrhea, anorexia, neuralgia, periodontal disease, deafness and shock. It kills bacteria, is antiviral, eliminates lung congestion, stops muscle spasms, lowers blood pressure, is immunomodulatory, aphrodisiac, antioxidant, a free radical scavenger, rejuvenative, circulatory, cephalic, nervine, tranquilizing, stimulant, decongestant, anti-rheumatic and memory boosting. Calamus has also been known to quite easily heal diabetes. In India, Calamus is known as Vacha, which means speech—and it alows direct expression and articulation of natural thought. It connects voice and heart, instills the ability to speak truth. Its specific connection is not just to the nervous system, but also the digestive, circulatory, respiratory, reproductive and lymphatic systems, and the adrenals. It is heating, awakens digestive fire and purges the orifices of the head of toxins—and has a special affinity for muscles and fat, reproductive tissues, nerves and plasma.

It has been used for the immediate removal of fatigue, Native Americans and settlers would chew on the root in order to work all day or run long distances—it increases energy and modulates hunger, giving vigor and willingness to continue. It restores and nourishes the entire body, strengthens, relaxes and stimulates at the same time, calms and centers. For learning, it stimulates attention and allows the up-take of knowledge. Calamus is very effective in bringing consciousness into the present, removing anxiety, and allowing focus to finally take place, naturally, without tension. In easing anxiety, it is in a class of its own. Calamus allows open awareness. Clarity. It unifies the body into one whole, better able to deal with tension and simply be present. It can clear post-traumatic stress disorder, remove panic, clear the mind and return to presence in the moment.

Large doses can easily overstimulate the stomach and result in vomiting. The traditional way of using Calamus is to chew on the root without swallowing the fibers, just the juices. Alternatively, you can make tea, or, after a while, if confident in your experience using the plant, you can also eat it after chewing. Being strongly antimicrobial, chewing on it can fight infections directly, or prevents catching contagious disease in the first place. Chew it around sick people and you won't get sick. It also gives vitality and keeps you pushing through whatever symptoms you may be experiencing. Calamus is an extremely powerful adaptogen, connecting most of the body's systems and strengthening them immediately, and in the long term, increasing the vital force in a mindful way and giving energy that can be used in the present, with clarity and courage.

Licorice

Licorice is a supremely balanced adaptogen that replenishes the full, deeply rooted energy of the body, no matter how it was lost in the first place—whether to exertion, stress, illness or aging, or anything in between. It's a perfect kidney tonic that creates balanced energy to support brain power, sexual health, the integrity of bones and the body's skeleton, and overall healing ability. It is widely used to heal backaches. It is also a strong lung tonic, uniting all the energies of the body and giving strong breath. It is the Universal Herb, working directly with the lungs, spleen and kidneys, balancing the five organs, strengthening the tendons, bones and muscles, growing muscles and giving strength everywhere, and healing wounds with internal or external application. It restores the adrenal glands, boosts moods and fights stress, stabilizes blood sugar, regulates the functions of the immune system and the hypothalamic-pituitary-adrenal axis, and soothes and heals the whole digestive system.

Licorice helps resist a wide array of bacteria, viruses and fungi. It stops diarrhea, clears heat and dispels toxins. It protects the liver, is anti-inflammatory, and stimulates the immune system when dealing with chronic disease and fatigue. Licorice also deals with diseases of the stomach, such as irritable bowel syndrome, inflammatory bowel disease, gastritis and ulcers.

Nettles

Nettle is a powerful blood purifier that improves the kidneys and heart, and removes toxins and metabolic wastes while cleaning out the intestinal tract and inducing a state of resilience in the entire body. It's an overall health tonic that is also used for headaches, internal bleeding, anemia, fatigue, high blood pressure, arthritis, skin inflammations, asthma, and a host of other problems. It's a perfect herb for chronic diseases requiring long term treatment, and beyond use for disease, it improves general health and functioning, being a nutritive herb, a gentle cleanser and detoxifier with a stimulating effect on the all-important lymphatic system. It also works as an adaptogen for the endocrine system, adrenals and the kidneys and restores all tissues and nutritive pathways, powerfully building the blood. Nettles build health and proper functioning, are very antioxidant and intensely nutritive, giving stable, balanced energy.

Nettles roots restores male sexual energy, and the seeds are very energizing and quick acting, restoring the kidneys and adrenals. Eating fresh seeds can cause powerful sensations of stimulation, while dried seeds are softer in action and more of an overall balanced adaptogen. They also give a sense of wellness and clarity, with stable energy levels throughout the day, increased effort capacity and reduced stress, and a tendency to rest and relax after effort, despite the stimulating effects. Nettle seed will remove deep fatigue and burnout, lack of focus, depression, anxiety and overall body pain, and restore the overall good functioning of the system. They can also improve mental balance, giving a focused sense of well-being and connectedness, and even joy, with a joy of effort and an increase and body-mind endurance. Seed doses are small, from just a pinch to a tablespoon, and the dose actually gets smaller over time, as one gains a connection with the plant. Nettle is a recognized adaptogen and an amazingly powerful ally for any human being.

Gentian

Yellow Gentian is an extremely powerful bitter tonic that gives the body fresh vigorous power and stimulates the digestive organs into vital action. It is also an antidote for the poisonous bites of insects and animals—or wherever poison may be involved. Traditionally, whenever there was cold in the body, with lack of vitality and ability to overcome conditions and disease, Gentian was given and it restored power. Even when faced with complete collapse, Gentian works.

It increases circulation and body temperature, increases assimilation of food, restores the body after fevers and any other kind of general depletion, is a stimulant, a powerful tonic and it increases appetite. It scavenges free radicals from the body, has been shown to increase natural endurance, resistance to effort and bacterial infection, viral infection, fungal infection, cancer and malaria. It also reduces liver damage. It also normalizes the function of gastric glands, immune function, allergic reactions, inflammation and blood pressure, blood sugar, and heals diarrhea and arthritis. Should not be used during fevers, or when there are ulcers, and in large doses it increases the pulse and can cause indigestion and vomiting.

It gives resistance to a wide range of biological conditions while normalizing the body's functions and improving vital power and energy. It increases resistance to toxins, protects the liver from chemical damage, and increases endurance and stamina, relieving fatigue - Gentian is a powerful adaptogen.

Red Clover

Red Clover is very common and very powerful. Back when tonics were popular, before antibiotics and modern medicine started destroying the health of the average human being, Red Clover was one of the most empowering, supportive, and easy to handle tonics available. Back then, people had to be well and stay well in order to work, and Red Clover was the herb they relied on to keep the body strong or quickly get it back to strength. In Europe, since beginningless time, Red Clover was the top plant for increasing resistance to disease and endurance to heavy work. It is a whole body tonic that simply gives power.

The traditional notion about Red Clover was that even if you were seriously ill —very seriously ill—it would bring you back to working condition. When the body was consumed, no matter what the various symptoms were, whether cancer or the flu or a nervous disorder, Red Clover would change the course of the situation. It is one of the best blood purifiers, especially for cancer, and a great tonic that produces healthy flesh, especially in the case of weakness or thinness. In China, as well, it is greatly esteemed as a tonic, and proven to kill viral and fungal infections.

It has been used to raise resistance to acute and chronic infections, to cancer, to tuberculosis, overworked nervous systems, loss of memory, senility, confusion, general mental failure and mental strain, and even beyond this, it was used to recover from a state of complete exhaustion.

In modern tests, Red Clover has been proven to increase resistance to bacterial infection, fungal infection, cancer, tumor formation, metastasis, viral infection, malaria, liver damage, free radical damage, and it also protects the skin against UV radiation.

Even in cancer patients nearing collapse, in centuries past Red Clover was found to stabilize the body and slow the progression of cancer.

It has a direct action upon the brain, improving its nutrition and resistance to any kind of failure, and it also connected the brain to the extremities—the hands and feet, and improves circulation there. Ultimately, it increases vital energy, and with it, the ability to fight any disease or condition, is recognized as an adaptogen, and is beyond any doubt an incredibly useful power herb that should be used by anyone.

Sarsaparilla

Sarsaparilla (Smilax ssp) was, in Native American culture, the supreme blood tonic, and they held that any weakness could be transformed into a strength by using Sarsaparilla. Whenever disease turned into general exhaustion without recovery—a state of decay and consumption, Sarsaparilla was the immediate remedy.

It is a general tonic, a metabolic stimulant, pituitary stimulant, immuno-stimulant, antibiotic, antiseptic, anti-inflammatory, testosteronic (it aids testosterone activity in the body), aphrodisiac, and much more. When someone needs to mount resistance to an infection, or even worse, is succombing to disease, the powerful life force building power of Sarsparilla comes into play, and it is useful for any other imaginable scenario that requires vitality.

Sarsparilla is used for resistance to chronic infection and autoimmune disease, as well as cancer. It can also grant recovery from a state of complete exhaustion, or utter lack of vitality caused by chronic disease. In the old days, someone suffering in the latter stages of Syphilis, with yellow skin, bony deposits, falling hair and insanity caused by nervous tissue breakdown, could still be returned to vitality and balance by taking Sarsparilla. In modern times, though mostly forgotten, it has been successfully used for autoimmune diseases like psoriasis (where it combines well with Burdock, Yellow Dock and Cleavers), and for rheumatoid arthritis. It is one of the most powerful adaptogens, with a powerful tonic effect that applies to all systems of the body and can balance or power through innumerable conditions—and has been revered as such by many cultures.

Burdock

Burdock is the true restorative and nourishing tonic, both reliable and subtle, stabilizing the constitution of the body and perfectly strengthening the assimilation, utilization and elimination of all substances. When used daily, it perfects the functioning of the entire being. It is a great metabolic tonic and blood purifier, working directly with the lymphatic and endocrine systems and improving the liver and kidneys.

Wellbeing is the playing field of Burdock, the restoration of balance and normality—it synchronizes all the body's organs and systems and perfects the metabolic balance through which nutrients and energy are used. It restores activity and vigor, increases secretions, cleansing and tissue feeding, and perfect the metabolic activity of the liver, balancing the anabolism of fat in the body, which normalizes sugar use. Due to its effect on fat and protein metabolism, and its slow, balanced power, the American Indians would consider it "bear medicine", an image that gives a sense of its strength. Burdock removes sugar imbalances and cravings, which are never true energy, and restores the normal function of sexual hormones, which depend on fat metabolism. It works in the endocrine systems of both men and women. Through similar mechanisms, it also fully empowers the health of the skin, and integrates the whole body into a primal state of health. It supports both the hard and soft structures of the body, its genetic material and various tissue essences, increases the lifeforce, and should be used both as a daily, life-long adaptogenic herb, and in recovery from chronic disease.

Angelica

Angelica Archangelica is one of the most revered herbs in traditional medicine, and its almost identical Chinese relative (Angelica Sinensis) is widely recognized as an adaptogen, being known as "female ginseng". European Angelica is not nearly as recognized nowadays, although it is probably more powerful. In China, all the Angelica species are used interchangeably, and all have been used historically to boost general health and improve resistance to infectious disease and disease in general, and the varieties present in Japan and America are also very similar in effect. In European medicine, it was considered one of the most powerful tonics. We will discuss Angelica Archangelica, which is one of the most supportive and useful adaptogens anyone can use, and a very powerful plant—the tiny carrot is one of it's relatives, but Angelica reaches 12 feet in height.

The Vikings used Angelica as a form of currency, and Iceland's first law book had special punishment for the theft of Angelica.
It is one of the few plants in Iceland that have made it through the last ice-ace, and the Vikings used it for support during harsh winters, for power and general healing, and for regaining strength after illness. If the Vikings decided they needed Angelica, so should you—it is an amazing balancing tonic that is perfect for dealing with harsh daily conditions and plenty of adversity. It has an overall strengthening and calming effect, improving the whole nervous system and the vital energy of the whole body, activating the immune system, and acting as an antidepressant. In Japan, it is seen as powerful tonic medicine that increases milk flow in the mother and sexual vigor in the father, is associated with longevity in harsh conditions, and was used against infectious disease. Incidentally, it was also used as protection from infectious disease everywhere else on the planet. In China, it is used for female health—hot flashes, dry skin, mood swings, irritability, memory loss—and it is seen

as the best herb for this. Women who want to avoid hormone replacement therapy stay young using Angelica, and it is an old verified belief that woman who take Angelica maintain their youth far longer. The wives of Emperors and all the imperial courtesans used Angelica, and it also kept away allergies and their annoying symptoms. In America, the native species is Purple Angelica, and the Native Americans used the root, stems, leaves and seeds as a general tonic, a superb stomach treatment, and a whole-body vitalizing treatment against chronic disease. Overall, they used Angelica for strength and vigor, and to combat any kind of chronic illness.

In Europe, it was said to defend the heart against all poisons, meaning all toxins and all disease, including the bites of rabid dogs and other poisonous animals. It was called a "counterbane", something that would counter any disease or problem, and Angelica tea was used against anything that threatened to attack the body. It was the best remedy against the plague, and against poison in general. Chewing it kept infectious disease away ("pestilential air"), and even after catching a disease, Angelica was able to drive it out directly through urine and sweat. It was seen as a whole-body health booster, and there is a historic notion that continuous use of Angelica leads to unbelievable longevity. A very old "fountain of youth" drink, Carmelite water, had Angelica as its main ingredient, alongside nutmeg, lemon and lemon balm. Invented by monks who then succeeded in living very long lives for generations, a long list of famous European characters used Carmelite water for longevity, relaxation, protection from poisons, neurosis and headaches. Since Angelica vitalizes the body at a primal, cellular level, and kills viruses, bacteria and fungi, along with strengthening all the body's systems, there is no surprise regarding this historical use.

Angelica increases nutrient absorption, stimulates appetite, normalizes hormone levels, kills infection, increases circulation, stimulates all the major body systems, increases the energy release from sugars and fats, and combats fevers, colds, the flu, infections, gastrointestinal disorders, respiratory disorders, cerebral diseases and nervous system dysfunction. It's a very powerful antioxidant and energy booster, that is also anti-tumor, anti-inflammatory, anti-bacterial, anti-viral and anti-mutagenic. It is a powerful body and skin detoxifier, and has topical antibacterial and antiseptic properties, healing skin directly. It's an aphrodisiac, antispasmodic, nervine, hepatic, stimulant, tonic, digestive and diuretic, that has also been used against arthritis, rheumatism, chronic colds, nervous headaches, toothaches, chronic fatigue, menstrual problems, anorexia, urinary diseases, anemia, diabetes, hepatitis, nephritis, circulatory problems, stomach cancer, indigestion, insomnia, and to stop bleeding. In fact, in modern studies, it has even been proven to reduce the risk of bone fracture in female athletes with irregular menstrual cycles, and in people taking steroids. It is an excellent long term circulatory tonic and improves the whole respiratory system, its coumarin content inhibits cancer, it can stop infectious fevers, typhoid fevr, malaria, acute febrile diseases, has been used against ulcers, gout, sciatica, chills, aches, pains and bites of all sorts, myalgia, neuralgia, general dislike of the cold, and women's problems such as PMS and amenorrhoea.

Angelica is, by excellence, the supreme balancing and soothing adaptogen.

Oatstraw & Oats

Oats are a nervous system food, all parts of the plant nourish, restore, support and empower the nervous system, the brain, and the whole body. For pure medicinal purposes, the plant is gather between the time the flowers emerge and the seeds are fully ripe—when you squeeze the plant a thick white sap emerges, which has the look and taste of mother's milk. This is the Milky Oat stage, and in this stage you can juice the Oats and drink the juice directly, or make a tincture out of the plant, which can then be used for a long time. If you harvest the plant at the Milky stage, then dry it, it turns into Oatstraw, a similar but perhaps less powerful medicinal herb. The Oat grains themselves—who knows—they are not much discussed in the herbal tradition, but probably maintain the full power of the plant and use it in a different manner. Oat grains are certainly an adaptogen, and a perfect food, but we will be discussing Milky Oats here.

Milky Oats is a great nervous system tonic, particularly when the body has to cope with stress in the present. Milky Oats builds strength and lifeforce over time, but also has an immediate restorative effect, fixing nervous breakdowns, depression, general weakness, exhaustion, shock, tremors, emotional instability and pain, shattered nerves, and drug withdrawal symptoms. It brings back peace, re-establishes tranquility, and takes away chronic anger. Milky Oats allows you to bounce back and regain primal elasticity and emotional wellbeing. It restores lost strength and abilities, rebuilds the whole nervous system, feeds the heart and endocrine system. It is in the union of these three systems that the power of Milky Oats is found. Heart palpitations, and emotional heart trouble, mental and physical exhaustion, inability to focus, all are absorbed back into the nutritive growth flow of the present, increasing nerve force, sedating pain, and permanently stimulating the balance and vitality of the body-mind.

It is great for physical and mental exhaustion from too much work, for chronic gastrointestinal problems, for internal cold, melancholia, morbid obsession or addiction, and particularly in the loss of unity between the nervous system and sexual energy. Milky Oats has a great affinity for the nerve structure of the genital organs, and brings them back in line with the body-mind.

When there is deep depression, darkness, exhaustion, anxiety, no perspective and no positive interests, and certainly no energy for growth, and a great baggage of loss and grief, Milky Oats can power through gently. This seems like a contradictory action, but when powering through gently, one is brought back into the present effortlessly, and issues are resolved. Milky Oats is not a sedative or stimulating, but it stabilizes and enhances. It is also the best remedy for having to deal with sudden loss, with death, with people going away because of cancer or unfortunate events. Milky Oats then balances and nourishes the mind back to life. In the extreme, Milky Oats is for someone who is so frayed and beyond repair that they cannot even receive a hug—they would need one, but they can't stand being touched.

Milky Oats has been recognized as an adaptogen, but it would be hard to describe its adaptogenic nature succinctly. It works by uniting body and mind through the nervous and endocrine system, bringing the heart and the nervous structure of the sexual organs back together, and nourishing absolutely everything.

Agrimony

Agrimony removes tension of body and mind. If you're denying your pain and tension, hiding it behind layers of concepts or false energy, and you cling to speed and danger, excess and irresponsibility, Agrimony is for you. It removes the inescapable condition of being stuck in "fight or flight" mode, that stimulants, drugs and alcohol can never get you out of, but only exacerbate. This is also the tension of work, of business and social hierarchy. As opposed to the gentle stopping breath of meditation, the tense breath is held painfully, and Agrimony releases this hold. This is an actual physical condition—the lack of breath, the restricted breath, which is a sign of pervasive tension and clinging through all levels of one's life.

Agrimony normalizes the breath, so it is an adaptogenic of the Air element, of the breathing apparatus and mental tension, and as such it cures chronic bronchitis, asthma and similar complains, much as it cures the mental aspects. It cures the worst of coughing.

The interplay of tension and relaxation is always felt in the liver and kidneys, and Agrimony balances circulation to and from the liver, removing tension and anger, and it is a good remedy for kidney pain, especially severe nephralgia. Agrimony works with the lungs, liver, kidneys, spleen, the brain and the nervous system, it is a hepatic, a bile stimulant and a bitter tonic, and it has a normalizing effect upon the entire body. It also stops profuse bleedings when taken internally, which is another aspect of its tension-normalizing abilities. It is a very complex herb that has deep mental effects and at the same time normalizes the mind-body connection in the whole body. Someone who doesn't understand the negative effects of tension, of breath restriction and of the generalized mind-body pain it leads to, cannot understand the restorative, adaptogenic effects of Agrimony—but it is, indeed, a recognized adaptogen, and would most benefit those who do not understand its effects.

True Solomon's Seal

True solomon's Seal (Polygonatum Spp) nourishes, balances, restores and makes present the whole musculoskeletal system. It's a tonic for both body tissues and energy, and has a deeply empowering effect on the mind and brain. It restores mental vitality and allows mental work endurance.

It tonifies the spleen and stomach, refreshes the lungs, lubricates the heart, builds the marrow and strengthens the kidneys, bringing the whole body together. In this, it stops all kinds of tissue wasting, loss of appetite, abdominal distension, head tension and weakness of the extremities. It's a sweet nutritive for the tendons and joints and balances all muscle and bone problems. It balances mucous tissues as well, so its activity is felt in the lungs, gastrointestinal tract and reproductive system. It has a tonifying effect on both male and female reproductive systems, and builds the essence of the body. It tonifies the heart and leads to recovery from long term chronic illness, and augments any other herbs it is combined with. It decreases negative feelings of hunger, increases resistance to temperature extremes, and makes all tendons and bones strong.

True Solomon's Seal unites the heart and brain and restores mental energy after prolonged effort. It is the herb of mental vitality, a strong mind potent that only takes a few weeks to fully show its effects. With Solomon's Seal, there is no mental breakdown, no emotional breakdown, but only concentration, focus, wakefulness, great memory, and balanced effort. It is an adaptogen and recognized as such, and in its full effect on the mind and musculoskeletal system, it makes for an incredibly power herb.

Borage

Borage is the adaptogen that gives birth to joy and merryment, exhilaration and gladness. It brings comfort to the heart, drives away sorrow, dullness and melancholy, stills any form of mental sickness, and enlivens the blood.
According to Pliny the Elder, Borage is Homer's Nepenthe, "that which chases away sorrow", the herb whose name literally means 'not-sorrow' or 'anti-sorrow, and brings about absolute forgetfulness. It revives the anxious and cheers the hard working, removes pensiveness and melancholy, works against fever, even against the plague, venomous bites, complete exhaustion of the vital force, rheumatism, and an incredible multitude of other ailments. The Romans mixed borage and wine before entering combat, for reasons that are quite obvious. Borage restores natural balance to the endocrine system and the adrenal glands, restoring the carefree presence that is the natural state of every being. It also works the nervous system, acting at its very top, where it meets the endocrine system, in the hypothalamus and pituitary glands. It perfectly purifies the blood, defends the heart from all fevers, being capable of removing heat born of systemic infection, viruses and poisons. It has been used for scarlet fever, contagious fevers, in all cases augmenting the vital force, as it "recreates the spirits, and gratifies or pleases the stomach".

When there is complete exhaustion and lack of spirit, Borage brings everything back up and puts it into play. Overthinking, over-arching stress, self-criticism, chronic disease and menopause, Borage health them, rebuilds the nervous system, the vital force, and restores natural mental presence.

Calendula

Calendula is cheerful and vibrant, a balancing tonic that supports the whole body and gently but powerfully feeds it. It also increases resistance to viral and bacterial infections, cancer and infected wounds. It grants resistance to a wide range of biological factors, is a very strong free radical scavenger and antioxidant, protects the guy, has anti-HIV activity, protects the mouth and teeth from decay, and reduces tumors. It also normalizes the immune function, inflammation, and closes chronic wounds. Both internally and topically, it is wound-healing and stops infection, being able to stimulate the immune system into healing, and specifically raising resistance to viral disease and infection both locally and in the whole body system.

It removes anger, frustration and irritability, and supports the liver and gallbladder, where these emotions originate. It is also great for ulcers and gut inflammation, and being anti-fungal, can normalize many intestinal problems, balancing intestinal flora, healing the gut wall, and bringing the immune system back into the interplay of gut and lymphatic system. Calendula powerfully supports the lymphatic system, which is why it heals the gut—the digestive, lymphatic and immune systems are deeply connected. If there is tiredness and fatigue, toxicity and low level infection that is generalized in the body, swollen glands and chronic issues, Calendula supports the entire healing and balancing process. It is traditionally seen as a powerful but gentle blood cleanser, and has been used in preventing and healing cancer. Calendula is not the most powerful herb for reversing states of complete exhaustion, but it does create lifeforce and balances the whole body. Where it excels is as an adaptogen in infections and wound healing, managing the entire immune system and all the systems that support it—and is recognized as such.

Dandelion

Dandelion, the tiny herb everyone ignores, happens to be one of the most appreciated ancient healing herbs, and a newly recognized adaptogen. It is one of the most powerful blood builders and purifiers, restoring and balancing the blood, and renewing energy and endurance. It has been used in Chinese medicine to increase the body's ability to resist disease and heal all of its systems—it works by detoxifying and purifying, removing all germs and toxins, and enhancing the immune system. To show the depth to which Dandelion works, it has been shown to increase the effectiveness with which the body remodels its own bones, and it can remove bone infections. If you suffer from chronic lethargy, dandelion will clear out your blood and stimulate energy.

Dandelion has shown anti-bacterial effects against many drug-resistant bacteria, including Staphylococcus aureus, as well as antiviral activity against the flu and other viruses. All the plant's parts are effective against all kinds of infections—hepatitis, respiratory infections, pneumonia, bronchitis, and so on. Dandelion works through the liver and kidneys, and clears heat and fiery toxins—that is, even the worst kind of viral toxicity manifested by certain infectious diseases. Toxic heat has the symptoms of red, swollen, painful eyes, and Dandelion is specifically good for this. Incidentally, these are also symptoms of virally toxic infectious diseases. Other historical uses in China, which have also been verified through government testing (well funded in that country), are for cancer, dermatitis, fever, inflammation, appendicitis, boils, abscesses, stomach aches, and snake and insect bites.

In the western world, Dandelion has been tested and proven to work against most cancerous cells, triggering cancer cell death even at lose-dose extracts. Further testing is ongoing and will likely prove the same effect for all cancer types. Dandelion has become a scientifically-proven, accepted natural anti-cancer agent, period.

Dandelion leaves they are 15% protein, and one cup of dandelion leaves contains 112% of the daily recommended vitamin A, 535% of vitamin K, and 32% vitamin C, among a host of beneficial chemicals, some of which are exclusive to Dandelion. It ranks as the 9th best food out of a wide variety of vegetables and grains. In a wide battery of tests in the eastern and western worlds, it has been shown to be a potent antibacterial and antiviral, anti-tumor, anti-cancer, anti-oxidant, a stimulant of positive internal bacteria, and an immense number of other benefits, that confirm its ancient use as an adaptogen and its modern ranking as such.

Wild Indigo

Wild Indigo stimulates the immune system and increases vital energy and lifeforce. Its close relative, Astragalus, has long been considered an adaptogen, and Wild Indigo is now also recognized as such. Its historical use is in treating all kinds of infectious disease, from digestive infections to fevers coupled with infection. It also stimulates the entire body to reach a new degree of health and escape states of chronic exhaustion—it was used to both increase resistance to epidemic disease and strengthen the body to survive any kind of diseased condition.

Wild Indigo has an antiseptic effect, both internally and externally, it powerfully stimulates the endocrine and nervous systems, cleans the lymphatic system, heightens liver functions, increases bile, removes infection from the blood, strengthens glands in order to resist toxins, and prevents colds. It was used to raise resistance to scarlet fever, typhoid infection, diphtheria, septic fever, malaria, variola, cerebrospinal meningitis, septic disease, intermittent fevers, tuberculosis and rheumatism. Wild Indigo was also used to powerfully break through states of deep exhaustion resulting from disease and acute infection, including the body's tendency to putrefy, open ulcers, lack of tonus and a tendency towards molecular death and decomposition, gangrene—and to recover from both the generalized exhaustion and the acute infection itself. It raises resistance to bacterial, viral and protozoan infection. On an even deeper level, Wild Indigo resists the toxic environment produced by infecting organisms, which release endotoxins that overwhelm the body's systems and cause generalized tissue breakdown. Wild Indigo can clear the toxic environment and resist the destruction of tissue. It it also useful in raising resistance to chronic infection, and has been tested as an immune stimulant, activating production and activity of phagocytes and lymphocytes, as well as containing compounds that increase resistance to tumors, cancer, free radical damage, hypertension, liver damage, hypoglycemia, mutagenicity and ischemia. Its antibacterial, antifungal and antiviral (shown to increase viral resistance to HIV, polio and herpes) effects have also been proven.

Wild Indigo is an adaptogen due to its whole body vitality empowering effects, and its wide ranging protective abilities, especially the union of nervous and endocrine systems resulting in resistance to generalized system toxicity born of bacterial endotoxin production. The more we are faced with antibiotic resistant bacteria, or with complex, mutating viral infections, the more valuable Wild Indigo and other adaptogens become. It is also valuable because it has specific compounds that show resistance to cancer, and wide resistance to infection. It is a dynamic system-wide antiseptic that clears the blood and strengthens the life-force of the body, while protecting tissue and having the power to resist even the most generalized states of weakness. In more normal conditions, it overcomes fatigue and weariness, and gives birth to a sense of vigor, perfect tone and wellbeing.

Black Cohosh

Black Cohosh is a strong tonic for the central nervous system and musculoskeletal system, a life-giving adaptogen that raises resistance to a large number of stressors, and is especially useful for the female body, female reproductive health, and additionally is great at healing arthritis. Black Cohosh normalizes the experience of menopause and the menstrual cycle, taking the variation and chaos out, and replacing it with an empowering, healing female energy.

The root was used by Native Americans to improve general health and the female reproductive tract—irregular menstruation, lack of strength, chronic coughing and poor digestion, and the general empowerment of the female body. Black Cohosh strenghtens the overall vital force, and the reproductive system then normalizes and reaches higher functioning. Menopause, irregular menstrual cycles, infertility and tendencies to miscarry were all healed with Black Cohosh. Estrogen affects the tissues of the female body, including nervous system functions, resulting in great emotional instability during menstrual cycles. Black Cohosh was the Native American tonic for dealing with PMS, and nervous troubles in general, including hysteria, for which it is a direct cure—slow but permanent. Formonentin, an isoflavonoid found in Black Cohosh, stimulates production of estrogen in the female body and also has anti-cancer and anti-fungal activity. The tonic power of the herb, along with the anti-cancer activity, can prevent uterine, breast and cervical cancer, and the fungicidal function is very useful in candida. The rhizome of Black Cohosh is used in hormone regulation—mood swings, hot flashes, irregular menstruation, pain or loss of menstruation, as a fertility aid, or in PMS. It has to be used for several cycles in order to normalize the functions of the cycle.

The root is an arthritis cure, and reduces inflammation and pain in chronic arthritis—whether it is osteoarthritis, where the pain results from wear and tear, or rheumatoid arthritis, where it is especially good because of the immune system involvement. Black Cohosh was considered absolutely effective in acute rheumatism, healing even the worst cases.

Its close relatives, Aconite and Anemone, are powerful painkillers, and Black Cohosh shares many of their traits. It also has a host of steroid-like substances that reduce inflammation both internally and topically. These two functions are, together with its general adaptogenic ability, at the root of its anti-arthritic potency. Overall, Black Cohosh is a tonic, adaptogenic, increases digestive secretions, has a tonic effect on mucous and serous membranes, is tonic to the kidneys, nervous system and the uterous, normalizes reproductive functions, increases digestive secretions, and much more, and has been used to treat acute rheumatism, malaria, tuberculosis, fevers, rheumatic fever, cerebral complications of fevers, bone infections, measles, small pox, asthma, cough, lung diseases, ulcers, disease symptoms that would today be called fibromyalgia, nervous dysfunction, epilepsy, nervous excitability, neuralgia, nervous inflammation, spinal inflammation, hysteria, rheumatic neuralgia and headaches, eye inflammation, congestion headaches, and a wide array of chronic diseases. This gives insight into its general power to heal. Black Cohosh was used to raise general resistance, strength and adaptability to a wide range of disease, and to recover from the complete state of exhaustion that would set in, complete with whole mind and body chronic symptoms. It raised resistance to acute viral, bacterial and parasitic and fungal infections, chronic infection, autoimmune disease of any kind, and to simply keep the body going through extreme conditions. It has been scientifically shown to resist all these kinds of infections, as well as cancer, tumors in general, protect from free radicals, protect the liver, normalize tension, temperature, inflammation, blood sugar, gastric dysfunction, edema, ulcers and hyperactive immune functions.

It is, ultimately, an adptogen that is specific to women, and to the female body and mind, that has an incredibly wide range of protective and resilience uses in the harshest inner and outer conditions, and that most specifically affects the nervous and musculoskeletal systems directly and profoundly. Its role in the estrogen cycle would probably make the modern man think twice before using Black Cohosh, but this is a reductive view—plants that regulate female energy make incredibly protective allies, and the Native Americans did not hesitate to use Black Cohosh. Especially when having to resist disease, its energy, different from that of more masculine plants, would be a tremendous complement.

Fenugreek

Fenugreek is rich in saponins that have a deep link to stimulating growth hormone release, and the pituitary gland in general. The pituitary is in many ways the master gland of the body, having a role in an endless number of body and mind processes. It regulates the adrenal glands, thyroid, ovaries and testes, and from each of these, a hormonal cascade is released and then cycled back into the pituitary. Fenugreek is a stimulant, anti-inflammatory, aphrodisiac, anabolic, anti-parasitic, hepatoprotective, and it has a general role in improving the vital force of the body, cell protection, and recovery from illness and infectious disease, particularly diseases that cause skin irritation, diabetes, fever, anorexia, swelling, burns, abscesses, ulcers, digestive issues, cough and bronchitis. It has been scientifically shown to be an aphrodisiac and to cause significant improvements in muscle strength, has been traditionally used as an adaptogen in China and India, is now recognized as such in the west, and its relatives, Astragalus, Wild Indigo, Red Clover and Licorice are all adaptogens. It has also been lab-tested against cancer, and proven to be toxic to a wide range of cancer cells, but empowering to normal body cells.

Fenugreek is an powerfully balancing herb that works directly on the hormonal system, the reproductive tissues, the blood and plasma, marrow and nerves, the respiratory and digestive systems, and the urinary and reproductive systems. In China it is used to treat weakness, anemia and impotence, and in India it is used for countless issues, as well as being a general tonic for good health. It is a strongly warming herb that gives strong energy and primal life-force, and rebuilds the lower body (where the urinary, reproductive and digestive systems are), reconnecting it to the upper body (respiratory system, marrow, nerves, pituitary gland), replenishing the whole body and its blood and plasma. Fenugreek is an adaptogen for power and it grows naturally on all continents.

Goldenseal

Goldenseal is the adaptogen for acute and chronic infections of the respiratory tract. It directly blocks the resistance capacity of bacteria, which, in a world that is more and more being threatened by antibiotic resistant bacteria, is a life-saving quality. Goldenseal is also a tonic—described as being mild, permanent and certain, having an inherent influence over the stomach and digestive organs, restoring tone to the stomach, acting as a general restorative, and removing all negative influences that result from an energetically unbalanced stomach, such as anorexia, indigestion and general weakness. It has been clinically used to increase resistance to all sorts of microbial infections (Streptococcus, Staphylococcus, tuberculosis, malaria and so on), and resistance to hyper and auto-immunity, which are actually the cause of death in Ebola and other killer viruses, by way of a cytokine storm, which is a hyper auto-immune reaction resulting in the immune system attacking its own body.

Goldenseal has been used as an adaptogen, an empowering tonic capable of plowing through the state of complete exhaustion that comes with chronic and acute disease, being able to normalize all functions of the body. It is now a recognized adaptogen. Because it is known to work against the flu, it has become very popular, and is now a threatened species in the wild, so if you choose to use it, make sure it has been grown commercially, not taken from the wild. Ultimately, Goldenseal is superb at protecting and normalizing the body, it is not as powerful at generating energy and lifeforce as the most powerful adaptogens are, but it restores and tonifies, balances and protects, and is able to remove bacteria directly and modulate the immune system so that it never turns against itself. These are all superb functions in the fight against the world's most dangerous diseases.

Astragalus

Astragalus root builds and restores the general health of the body, especially adrenal fatigue. It is useful againstfibromyalgia and chronic fatigue syndrome, or for people who are simply run down and getting frequent colds, or have seasonal allergies.

It increases cell growth and cell longevity, and stimulates antibodies, is a tonic for the heart, lungs, liver and kidneys, lowers blood pressure, increases circulation, and also stimulates interferon, which keeps viruses from multiplying. It is great at increasing the lifeforce energy of the body, helps regulate stress and immune functions, and has been used against chronic auto-immune disorders, mononucleosis, Alzheimer's, cancer, hepatitis, asthma, arthritis, and for broken bones.

Astragalus gives movement energy and protective energy, improves the mononuclear phagocyte system of the immune system, it stimulates pituitary-adrenal cortical activity and renews red blood cells in the bone marrow. It is a supportive adaptogen that has an upwards, energizing function, and renews energy and protective functions. I include it here because, although it is a Chinese herb, it can be easily grown in the Western world.

Eleuthero

Eleuthero, also known as Siberian Ginseng, is the first adaptogen identified in Russia, as part of Russia's intensely government sponsored search for a perfect category of stimulating and balancing plants that would be applicable to performance in any aspect of life. That point in space and time is also the origin of the term adaptogen. Eleuthero has since been used by Russian athletes and astronauts, as well as for civilian and military performance of all kinds, and has always provided exceptional results. It increases physical endurance without any added heat, aids recovery and fatigue, strengthens the immune system, reduces stress, increases energy and vigor, strengthens the skeleton and tendons, and is a long term stimulating and restorative agent for the whole body and mind. It increases both focus and relaxation, balances moods and improves sleep patterns. It also improves the balance of neurotransmitters, those noted in studies being dopamine, serotonin, norepinephrine, and epinephrine, which makes it an excellent mind tonic. It doesn't overstimulate, and it modulates the nervous, endocrine and immune systems. Because of the plant's popularity, a lot of extracts are fakes, so it is better to use the herb directly.

Rhaponticum

Rhaponticum, known as Maral Root, is the second of the Russian adaptogens. It is a mind-body stimulant that improves memory and learning, the work capacity of the muscles and skeleton, and anabolic and adaptogenic processes. It increases muscle mass, powers the heart, stimulates the immune system, improves blood circulation in the brain and muscle tissues, elevates primal lifeforce, regulates blood sugar, restores and regenerates the entire body, improves the mind—focus, concentration and mental endurance, reduces depression, increases resistance to colds, sexual energy, and overall strength and energy. It's a well known adaptogen that works in a very straightforward, empowering manner, and has always been used as part of Russian adaptogenic formulas, because it increases work capacity in all ways and helps the body adapt and recover when faced with a large number of external stressors. Anti-cancer, anti-microbial, anti-fungal, and anti-parasitic, strongly antioxidant, and significantly modulates cellular activity and DNA replication.

Rhodiola

Rhodiola, know as Golden Root, is the third Russian adaptogen, which has wide and balanced effects on the immune system, protects the adrenals and the heart, enhances brain function, reduces cortisol and stress, fatigue, and is a mild nervous system tonic. Golden Root protects from temperature extremes, balancing the body's response to both hot and cold weather, modulates the use of oxygen at a cellular level, increases strength and endurance, and reduces recovery time after effort or stress. Its effects on stress are powerful, on both mental and physical levels, improving mood and focus, reducing depression, and behaving like a general tonic for the whole body. Studies show Golden Root to be equal in effect to many anti-anxiety and anti-depression drugs, but without any of the side effects, and all the positive effects of an adaptogen that works directly with the lifeforce and protective, resilient strength-energy of the body.

Turmeric

Turmeric is India's main spice, and top all-around medicinal herb. It is used there as an adaptogen, having been proven both in use and studies to be incredibly useful in an immense range of diseases. The same range and depth of use is now being proven by Western studies, with over 600 studies now backing its effects. It is one of the strongest antioxidants on the planet, with a wide, balancing antioxidant effect on all the body's tissues, and an increase in the body's ability to defend itself on a cellular level by producing its own internal and specific antioxidants. Turmeric reduces inflammation both immediately and long term, by modulating stress related inflammation. Its anti-inflammatory effects are broad spectrum, and specifically protect from internal or external heat-shock. Turmeric is strongly antiviral, anti-bacterial, anti-fungal and anti-cancer. It has been tested as having extensive effects against a large variety of viral, bacterial and fungal threats, as well as cancers.

Turmeric directly heals the liver and improves its functioning, protects the stomach and ends digestive disorders, arthritis, asthma, and eczema, protects the heart, relieves nausea, and is a specific for wounds and skin problems. It heals skin ulcers, itching, psoriasis, insect stings, ringworm, snakebites, herpes cuts, measles, chickenpox, and anything else. It is effective against diabetes, allergies, Alzheimer's, and chronic disease in general, which it removes through regulating growth factors, cytokines, enzymes and various transformation factors of the body. Through topical application, it heals bone inflammation, bruises, sprains and even breaks.

India's medical tradition holds Turmeric to be an adaptogen, one of a few herbs that are known in India to work deeply on an inter and intra-cellular level, able to block the growth and effects of invading pathogens while empowering the body's own cells and processes. In the Western world, science has proven Turmeric's effect against all kinds of cancer and viruses, including HIV, HPV, herpex simplex, and the deadly Rift Valley Fever virus. It is impossible to clearly pin-point Turmeric's adaptogenic behavior, and one must simply go back to the Indian understanding that it does its work on the most subtle cellular level, and all its endless effects stem from there.

Ginger

Ginger is another Indian herb that is seen as a spice in the Western world, but recognized as a deep cellular adaptogen in Ayurveda. Ginger is an incredibly warming herb that uplifts the spirit. In this phrase lies the key to its understanding—it works by warming and tonifying everything on a cellular level, and the empowering vigor that results is carried and balanced all the way into the mind. Ginger clears and stimulates the mind, vitalizes the circulatory system, strengthens the stomach, removes all nausea, and modulates inflammation causing genes.

It is immunostimulant, and taken together with Turmeric is a great defense against any kinds of infections. Ginger has also demonstrated anti-cancer activity in the lab, thins the blood, and despite its great warmth, can have an overall cooling effect on the body. It moves fluids through the cartilages and joints, and soothes tense muscle. It opens the skin to release toxins and cold, re-starts activity, improves fat metabolism and bile secretion.

Traditionally, it has been used to strengthen mothers during labor and delivery. This is enough detail about its uses, ultimately, it's a very warming and stimulating mind-body adaptogen that works on the deepest level. In the Western world, the Indian herb Ashwaganda is seen as an adaptogen, while Ginger, Turmeric and Cinnamon are mere spices. Ayurveda, however, holds these to be superior to Ashwaganda, as adaptogens, due to their ability to protect and empower cells, the nervous system and gene expression in a primal manner.

Cinnamon

Cinnamon is warming, improves circulation, digestion, blood sugar, thins blood, and has such a deeply tranquilizing effect on the central nervous system that it has been shown to be able to balance the stimulation of methamphetamine. In other (sadly cruel) tests, it has delayed convulsions and death in animals injected with a strychnine (poison) overdose. Just this much fully proves its status as a highly potent adaptogen that connects the nervous system strongly to the circulatory system and the body's other functions. Cinnamon also regulates temperature, adrenal tension, and has a very strong antibiotic effect against a wide array of bacteria and fungi. It is also deadly to viruses of all kinds, having been shown to neutralize viruses very fast. Studies on Cinnamon's effect on Avian Flu H9, HIV, Herpex Simplex all showed it to be very effective, not only killing viruses but also helping the body develop immunity. Not surprisingly, it is also anti-parasitic.

Cinnamon has also been shown to treat asthma, diabetes, menopausal problems, headaches, digestive disorders, impotence, bad breath, anemia and intestinal infection. Yes, it does do all this, mostly because it enhances overall fire in the system, from the deep level of the central nervous system, in union with the circulatory system. It releases anger and dependence, boosts memory power, cognitive skills, reduces mental fatigue, tension, depression and anxiety, and generally balances the gut and the head. It also supports the heart and boosts sexual energy—so it is a powerful full body adaptogen that has its roots in the primal heat of the nervous system.

Brahmi

Brahmi is part of a triad of Ayurvedic mind-herbs, and perhaps the most mental of them. The other two are Holy Basil and Calamus, which, having been used by many cultures, is not exclusive to India. Brahmi is a great tonic for the mind—improving clarity, cognition, memory and overall mood—it modulates neural activity to induce a state of positive relaxation, contentment and emotional stability, while connecting heart and mind and improving the functioning of neurotransmitters. It protects and strengthens nerves and the cerebro-spinal fluid, allows consciousness to recognize itself directly, promotes stable inner joy, and leads to the generalization of a subtle state that is similar to the relaxation of deep sleep or meditation.

Brahmi can regenerate brain tissue, and has been show to have a positive effect against Alzheimer's. It is also effective in letting go of opioid dependence—

which is a modern problem due to the prevalence of pain-killers. It modulates autoimmune response and body and brain inflammation, modulates blood pressure, is a strong antioxidant, is antimicrobial, and has been tested as a full-body adaptogen, showing its ability to fully stimulate and restore the lifeforce and energy of the system.

It has also been shown to modulate microcirculation, which is the blood's circulation through the very smallest blood vessels within organ tissues and the skin. Through its effect on micro-circulation, Brahmi improves the body's ability to directly heal, feed and improve itself—and Brahmi has been shown to be able to restore damaged nerves, which is notoriously hard to do. But this is all understood by Ayurveda, as Brahmi is one of the herbs traditionally held to be able to affect deep changes at a cellular level. It is a full mind-body adaptogen that works in subtle but direct ways to improve the balance, energy, integrity and function of the system. While it is not as stimulating to the lifeforce and energy as other adaptogens are, it is intelligent and creates long term improvements and immediate resilience on a deep level.

Holy Basil

Holy Basil (Ocimum sanctum—Tulsi) is also called the Queen of Herbs, The Incomparable One and The Mother Medicine of Nature. It's an all around adaptogen, an adrenal adaptogen, digestive tonic, antibacterial, antioxidant, antiviral, immune modulator, anti-inflammatory, anesthetic, and cell regenerator. It is traditionally considered a panacea, a heal-all, and looking at its uses, you realize it's a tonic for more or less all of the body's systems. Its use in India is for a mix of mental and body health and rejuvenation, as well as fevers, colds, coughs, indigestion, asthma and fatigue. It works directly on a cellular level, repairing and regenerating cells, and it actively scavenges free radicals from the heart, liver and brain.

It has the ability to clear the mind, restore and balance the adrenals, manage cortisol, overall stress and blood pressure. It boosts energy but is not a stimulant, so it can be used at night, and it supports the full sleep cycle. Like Brahmi, it revives nerves and strengthens the cerebro-spinal fluid, and can lead to a state of continuous awareness of consciousness, inner joy, and subtle generalized state of active relaxation akin to meditation and deep sleep.

Holy Basil also treats allergies, infertility, diabetes and radiation poisoning, and it does so by spontaneously mixing antibacterial, antiviral, antioxidant, anti-aging, anti-inflamatory, anti-arthritic and anti-stress functions. Its pain reducing abilities have been compared to modern painkillers by several studies.

The effect of Holy Basil is described as transforming the substances of the body into an essence that is stored in the heart and controls all other mind-body processes. This is a correct path of spiritual transformation, and Holy Basil can indeed transform tissues in this way, which is the opposite of the effect that stress and disease have on the body. This is why the herb is so revered in India.

Basil

Basil (Ocimum basilicum) is warming and drying, stimulating strong energy, and removing cold. Basil has been used to fight fatigue, loss of concentration, migraines, colds and coughs, bronchitis, infectious disease, insomnia, and anxiety and depression. It's a restorative tonic, a refreshing and uplifting antidepressant, with purifying and fortifying abilities. It works with the stomach, lungs, the adrenal cortex, immune, nervous and circulatory systems, the skin and women's reproductive system.

It stimulates the lungs and improves the ability of the lungs to use energy, removing fatigue, lack of vitality and depression. It also eases mental concentration, and has antioxidant, anti-cancer, anti-viral, and anti-microbial properties. It treats colds, flus and digestive disorders, and has been shown effective against multidrug resistant bacteria. Basil boosts the activity of neutrophils, which are the white blood cells that fight off viral infections. It can also remove symptoms of food poisoning, diarrhoea, stomach infections and vomiting.

It's a circulatory stimulant for the mind, and a nervine tonic, making the mind clean and clear, and it balances the release of cortisol, managing stress and re-setting sleep cycles and general moods.

Basil is full of active flavonoids, which protect the body at the cellular level, protecting both cells and DNA from radiation and free radicals. Its volatile oils protect from numerous bacteria, even after they have manifested resistance to common drugs. Basil also works as an anti-inflammatory by reducing the same enzymes that medicines such as ibuprofen do.

Ultimately, is western Basil an adaptogenic herb? This is up to you to determine from the evidence provided—it certainly affects a large number of body systems and provides protection in countless ways, to both mind and body, in ways similar to its adaptogen-proven Indian relative. Western Basil has unfortunately not undergone the same testing, and it is unlikely it will very soon, but in ancient medicine treaties it was called the King of Herbs, so even if you're using Holy Basil (the Indian variety), you should also take Western Basil.

Cayenne

Cayenne—is the most useful and direct central nervous system stimulant, a pure, energetic and permanent stimulant. Stimulation is key to healing, and cayenne is key to energy, the purest and the best herbal stimulant. It normalizes blood flow in the whole body, including the extremities, and has a very strong effect in the heart —an immediate ingestion of Cayenne at the beginning of a heart attack can completely stop it and remove symptoms. Ingestion of Cayenne at any time during and after a heart attack also does immense good—it immediately strengthens the heart, nerves, capillaries and arteries and provides relief. It stimulates the circulatory and digestive systems, and it does so in union with the nervous system. It rebuilds tissue in the stomach and heals intestinal and stomach ulcers, cleanses the blood fully, and helps heal arthritis and rheumatoid arthritis. Whatever herbs are used together with it, it is a catalyst for them, carrying their effects wherever they are needed most in the body. It removes colds and keeps them away, improves anyone's vitality, at any age, but is especially useful for old people, because it improves their vitality, activity and body head. It removes fatigue, loosens joints, and induces relaxation in the whole body.

When faced with the state of full exhaustion generated by chronic disease, Cayenne sustains the nervous system, steadies all other systems and allows sleep and relaxation. It heals the digestive system, marked depression and weakness, helps in acute fever, and stabilizes delirium. Cayenne resists and heals the putrid tendencies the body develops during complete exhaustion. It can be applied topically to ulcers and is tremendously effective when directly applied to toothaches. Cayenne powder applied to a wound immediately stops bleeding—internally, it balances pressure and stops hemorrhaging. In cancer studies, almost complete elimination of prostate cancer was shown, and Cayenne causes cell death in all cancers. It literally causes cellular destruction of cancer cells, because it directly feeds body cells through its nervous-blood systems union, while removing nervous support and blood flow to cancer cells. In fewer words, its pure and energetic heat manages to infiltrate malignant cells directly, while giving full resistance to body cells.

Cayenne is the adaptogen of the blood and nervous system. Every cell depends on blood supply, and on the coordination of blood and nerves. This is even more important in bone marrow cells, upon which the immune cells depend, and in the cells of the endocrine system, which Cayenne purifies and normalizes. It works on a primal, fundamental level, and builds lifeforce, resistance and energy.

Hawthorn

Hawthorn is a powerful heart tonic, improving the cardiovascular system's vitality and power, improving metabolic processes in the heart, managing blood pressure, and making the heart more resilient. Hawthorn removes depression and gloomy states by sheer heart power, increases general strength and well being, and strengthens the actual heart tissues. It is calming to the central nervous system, and stabilizes anxiety, nervousness, stress and irritability. It also protects arteries and blood vessels. While Hawthorn is not going to be recognized as an adaptogen very soon, because it doesn't have a measurable external effect, it has the ability to power the heart and blood and fully contain their effects into a strengthening internal balance—this is its adaptive value. When heart-blood is powerful, all other stresses and herbs can fall into place safely, without worry. An inner heart tonic is a very powerful adaptive force that should be a lifelong companion. Both the fruits and the leaves can be used. The more effort and stress you undergo, the more energy you need to use in order to maintain your focus and performance, the more important it is the have powerful heart-blood. Intense athletic exertion of the body and continuous mental concentration both put a tremendous amount of stress on the heart, and depend on the heart's presence and health. Long term progress in mental and physical activities, and long term growth of the body's health and resilience—both depend on the heart's full presence. Hawthorn is food for the heart, giving it power and protecting it from potential damage. It increases the force of myocardial contraction and the coronary blood flow, increasing cardiac output but having a beneficial effect on the heart. The heart works better, more powerfully, not harder, and in time it grows and supports the body even more.

Another herb that has deep affinity for the heart is Motherwort, and it can be used as a female herb-complement to Hawthorn. Motherwort fully gladdens and relaxes the nervous system and heart, which gives full relief for nervous sickness of all sorts, and elevates moods. It also gives energy and takes away anxiety, fatigue and unites the spine and heart—the nervous system and its center. I won't go into deeper explanations of this herb here, but you can use it together with Hawthorn. A third herb that is specific for the heart is Linden. Linden is tranquilizing and anti-spasmodic, removing tension and headaches, soothing the mind and letting cognitive processes flow. It kills fear, nervousness, colds and fevers, high blood pressure and emotional issues. It is relaxing to the heart, helping its arteries unwind and release tension. It manages blood pressure, is antiviral, and can be used externally to cure wounds.

Rosemary

Rosemary is probably furthest from most people's minds when picturing adaptogens—yet this common culinary herb has powerful effects on blood circulation and the nervous system. It increases blood flow to the brain, improving clarity and cognitive processes, lowers cortisol and stress, balances the adrenals, generating energy and good mood. It also stimulates nerve growth and repair, and is an adaptogen for the nervous system, able to remove the effects of toxins on the central nervous system. It has a radiant and uplifting mental effect, is tonic and restorative to the whole body, but especially to the nervous system, stimulates the liver and gallblader, controls blood pressure, muscle pain, colds, skin inflammation, breathing difficulties and headaches, is antibacterial, antiviral and anti-fungal, and it improves the energy processing of the while body.

People suffering from sciatica and neuralgia have been quickly benefited by Rosemary, and those are two example of chronic diseases that would benefit from the general and specific restorative abilities of this adaptogen. Rosemary is also specific for the heart, because it, just as Cayenne does, unites the nervous and circulatory systems.

Pine

The Pine is obviously adaptogenic in nature—a huge tree that stays green in a range of harsh climates, from -50 to +40 degrees Celsius, and whose every edible part is chock full of aromatic oils and other interesting chemical compounds. The needles of the Siberian Red Pine has been studied by Russians—who else—for its adaptogenic effects, and found to be a modulator of the immune system and general physical and mental stressors. Trials involving athletes, mothers, schoolchildren, and working people showed increased energy levels, endurance and reduces fatigue. Russian research from the 1930's had already shown that Pine needles contain what was called, at the time, "live elements", which allow them to sustain various extremes, and which are almost identical to health-supportive elements found in human blood. The Pine needle "live elements" were found to be easily and directly absorbed by the human body. During the 900 day Siege of Leningrad—this being World War 2—the city's population survived (in the sense that only a large minority died) on one 75 gram piece of bread per day. This bread was actually made of sawdust and food-grade cellulose, with added Pine needle extract. The one glass of water per day that Leningrad's citizens were allowed was also enriched with the extract. This is a verifiable historical fact. A topical paste called Conifer Green Needle Complex was developed by the Russian military, and it was used to heal burns, wounds and frostbite. After the war, the extract was further tested, and found to be anti-microbial, anti-viral and antifungal both internally and externally. The needles were found to be very rich in enzymes, sterols, hormones, di- and tri- terpenes, long chain high molecular alcohols and fatty and resin acids. The extract was said to promote quick recovery form viral infections, normalize the digestive system and protect the liver. More recent studies have shown Pine Needles to have strong antioxidant, antimutagenic, and antiproliferative effects on cancer cells. Different species of Pine have different components, but all species are extremely bio-active, in a minimalist, adaptive manner. And this is exactly the advantage of the Pine—it is simple, yet thrives.

Pine Pollen is even more powerful, it is hormonally balancing, estrogen-clearing, and testosteronic in a balanced manner that is useful to both men and women. Pine Pollen is a direct brain food that protects the liver, the cardiovascular system, generates glutathione—the body's master antioxidant, improves endurance, modulates immunity and the androgenic-estrogenic balance, is an aphrodisiac, and decreases DNA mutation. The best part is that, while Pine Pollen sounds somewhat exotic, it is almost as easily picked in the wild as Pine Needles are. It grows abundantly in small cone-like structures, which are the male Pine cone. Pine Pollen contains 80 ng/g of testosterone, 110 ng/g of epitestosterone, and 590 ng/g androstenedione, which can all be directly absorbed simply by keeping the pollen inside the mouth for a few minutes before swallowing—hormones and other subtle molecules permeate the mucous membrane of the mouth. An adaptogen of the nervous and endocrine systems, Pine is one of the most common food sources on earth, and one that has historically risen to the challenge and kept entire populations alive during the worst of times.

Periwinkle

Periwinkle is a mental adaptogen and mild stimulant. Its complex indole alkaloids, such as the much-researched vincamine, are abundant in all parts of the plant. It has been used to treat dementia and arterosclerosis, to stop internal bleeding and heavy menstrual bleeding. Applied directly to wounds, it is healing—which is a good sign of its adaptive power, as Periwinkle is used almost exclusively to increase cerebral blood flow and improve memory, focus and general peak brain function over long periods. It is very efficient and protective in this, and its specific connection to the brain, when taken in context of its ability to heal tissues directly, is very auspicious. Periwinkle also increases oxygen and glucose supplies in the brain, improves memory, has been used to treat senility and dementia in modern times, improves nutrient use by the brain, and is useful for recovery from strokes.

Black Cumin

Black Cumin increases energy, fatigue recovery, reduces depression and lack of vitality, and is a stimulant and tonic to the whole mind-body system. This is how the Ancient Greeks saw it, and their use of Black Cumin is mirrored in Indian medicine. Modern medicine considers is a potent antioxidant, anti-carcinogenic and anti-mutagenic, with the power to kill cancer cells directly through several molecular pathways. It also acts in preventing cancer, improving the body's defense system, a function which mirrors its ancient use as an all around strengthener and resistance builder. All studies done on it have confirmed its strong anti-cancer activity. Beyond being able to kill all types of cancer, it is effective in diabetes, asthma, kidney disease, cardiovascular disease, immune-system disorders, allergies, skin problems, fever, paralysis, anorexia, abdominal disorders, diarrhea and hemorrhage.

Black Cumin has a stabilizing effect on the central nervous system, is gastroprotective, antioxidant, anti-inflammatory, antitumor, antidiabetic, antimicrobial, anticonvulsant, modulates the immune system, prevents anxiety and depression, protects the liver and kidneys, improves respiratory health, intestinal health, fights skin conditions, is anti-parasitic, modulates neurological disorders (neuropathy, paralysis, etc), modulates insulin, can induce menstruation, relieves vomiting, kills parasites and intestinal worms, flushes body toxins, protects in the chronic stages of fever, relieves pain, headaches, tooth aches and conjunctivitis. Finally, it is a strong antibacterial (effective against a host of drug-resistant bacterial infections) and powerful antiviral—and restores the body after infection, having been shown to normalize red and white blood cell count, platelets and albumin, while modulating the immune system (it induces interferon production) and killing viral infections. It inhibits the factors that trigger a cytokine storm, which is the body's immune system turning against itself in the final stages of an acute viral infection—this being the mechanism of death in Ebola. It stimulates the production of bone marrow and immune system cell, protects normal cells from viral damage, and increases the number of antibody producing B cells. Black cumin also kills parasites and has been shown to increase testosterone levels, even within a system taken over by diabetes.

Black Cumin is obviously a very powerful adaptogen, thought to be a cure-all in several cultures—it enhances general well being, strength, boosts the vitality-energy and lifeforce of the body, and balances the body's systems while raising resistance to external threats. Beyond the modern proof of its power to resist disease, it is a brain tonic that improves intelligence and deeply strengthens the nervous system, acts as a natural aphrodisiac, improves eye health and vision, all of which, together with its deep black color, suggest an affinity for the mind and its natural adaptive powers, the brain's neuro-electrical play, natural enthusiasm, communication, inspiration, and the coordination of ideas and mental elements.

Cumin

Cumin the more common and available relative of Black Cumin, is perhaps not as powerful, and has not been studied as much, but shows adaptogenic functions nonetheless. It is also related to the mind, found to increase intelligence, eyesight, strength and immunity, is one of the best digestive tonics, removes toxins, improves absorption of nutrients, is an aphrodisiac and resists fever. It's also a remedy for headaches and removes mental and physical exhaustion, having a restorative effect on the body. It's a powerful nervine that has been used to treat epilepsy and tremors, and due to its antibacterial and antiviral functions, it's used as an adaptogenic tonic. In India, a very strong tea made from Cumin seeds is called Jeera water, and is used to improve heart health, cognitive functions, heal the eyes and strengthen the entire body.

Alfalfa

Alfalfa is a calming nutritive herb that fully supports the nervous system. Alfalfa is strongly alkaline, and removes all the stress related acids that are massively overproduced in a fatigued body. Alfalfa removes nervousness, and is a great restorative tonic, without acting as a stimulant. It improves the lifeforce, energy and vitality of the whole body, rejuvenating it and bringing its ability to grow and be resilient back into the present. When there is depression, loss of flesh and of the qualities of the body, digestive trouble, general weakness, anemia, nervous instability and lack of nutrient assimilation, Alfalfa empowers the kidneys and the nervous system and makes the body whole again. It improves the functional action of the brain and spinal cord, rebuilds teeth, cleans the blood and kidneys, and grants endurance and energy. For those dependent on tea and coffee, Alfalfa tea is a superior replacement, and takes away the nervous system's addiction to these stimulants.

One historically reported case, from a much less fortunate time, tells of a family in which seven children had died around the age of eighteen from an unknown disease that simply caused their emaciation. The last remaining child, a girl, started showing the same symptoms, but was given Alfalfa seed tincture. Her disease disappeared, and she went from 99 pounds to 133, completely regaining her health. Alfalfa is a strong adaptogen for balancing the nervous system and body, increasing the essential vitality of the kidneys and lower body while fully feeding the brain. It is a nutritive adaptogen, increasing vitality and strength directly, in a calm, restorative and empowering manner, and once strength is regained, energy, endurance and resistance to external factors all increase.

Thyme

Thyme is strongly antiseptic anti antimicrobial—being antiviral, antibacterial and anti-fungal. It eliminates toxins and boosts the entire immune system. It helps form white blood cells, boosting direct resistance to infection, and has been used to regain strength after illness, depression and chronic exhaustion. It revives, strengthens, and balances both mind and body, modulates blood pressure, stimulates circulation, increases concentration, intelligence and memory. It is antirheumatic and antiarthritic, and diuretic—helping flush out toxins from the body. It tonifies and strengthens the lungs, heart, circulatory, digestive and nervous systems, the muscles and skin, and directly boosts and modulates immunity. Additionally, a recent study has found Thyme to be more effective at pain reduction than ibuprofen, one of the most used over the counter pain medicines. Thyme is a good internal and external antiseptic, and can be used directly on wounds and sores to remove infection. It is an adaptogen and a very common and easily acquired power herb, extremely useful in preventing colds and infections of the respiratory tract, as well as overcoming them. This makes it an invaluable plant in the wake of the threat of rapidly spreading infectious disease.

Herb Collections

Herbs for the Mind

Sage significantly improves memory and immediate recall. It stops breakdown of acetylcholine, an essential neurotransmitter, and has been seen as a brain tonic and mind enhancer for ages.

Clary Sage leads to energized relaxation, stimulating and calming at the same time. It connects directly to the mind and sometimes gives vivid dreams.

Turmeric is a body protector by excellence, but it is also a whole-brain protector, in more ways than could ever be counted in a book.

Anemone grounds the mind, giving it solid stability and a good basis upon which to grow. It can reduce trauma and stabilize someone who is under the influence of drugs.

Periwinkle improves transport of oxygen and nutrients to the brain. It improves memory and cognition, and helps in cases of senility and dementia.

Rosemary improves recall and concentration, and physically, it increases blood flow to the brain, strengthens the heart and circulatory system, and inspires action and motion. It is an all-around brain tonic and nervine that lessens stress and depression while increasing alertness and memory. It is also one of the best tonics of the central nervous system, is a brain stimulant that increases intuition, clarity and positive attitude. It also stimulates cellular metabolism.

Peppermint stimulates and enlivens the mind, boosting creativity, energy, and the will to learn. It clears the connection between the brain and spine, stabilizes the body's winds and digestive processes, evening out the flow of energy in mind and body. It is an anti-spasmodic and clears out anger, balancing all the fluids of the body—blood, lymph, tissues, and spinal and cerebral fluids. Additionally, it opens the energy channels.

Basil eases mental fatigue and sharpens focus.

Oats balance the nervous system, restore and nourish it, ground the mind and protect brain tissue while granting concentration power.

Roses feed the nervous system, brain and heart, calming and centering emotions and spirit.

Lavender lifts depression and stress, and has a tranquilizing effect. It reduces irritability and anxiety, balances hormones, stimulates the immune system and has a protective, anti-bacterial effect. It removes scattered excess energy, anger and inflammation, and calms the heart-mind connection, balancing the sympathetic and parasympathetic nervous systems.

Skullcap is a wonderful nervine, nourishing the nervous system and brain, removing depression and pain, and sedating while at the same time improving concentration and attention.

Chamomile is a mild sedative and relaxant that brings emotions into natural centered focus, balancing body (solar plexus) and mind. It has been historically used to cure nightmares, addiction, and prolong life. Chamomile is an all-around relaxing herb that restores and balances everything, inducing patience, clearing heat and negativity, and restoring the liver and gall bladder.

Brahmi is an adaptogen with profound mental effects. In India, it is one of the three great herbs for the mind. In modern tests, it has been shown to increase memory and learning, decrease stress, to enhance the nervous system, reduce depression, have antimicrobial and analgesic effects, and to improve the complete adaptive ability of the whole body-mind system.

Holy Basil (Tulsi) is another adaptogen with deep mental effects, or rather, a mind enhancing herb with whole body adaptive effects. Tulsi protects the whole body from colds, protects the kidneys, heart and head, and cleanses the digestive and respiratory systems, while giving a sense of purity and lightness.

Calamus is the herb that fully clears the mental channels and enables expression, presence, mental and physical endurance, and a sense of natural awareness and well-being.

Wood Betony (Stachys officinalis) is a nervine tonic, a gentle acting herb that nourishes and builds vital energy over time. It connects the head and solar plexus and releases instincts and frees energy, while pacifying and stabilizing the mind, and being the go-to remedy for headaches.

Angelica is a calming tonic—a revitalizing and restorative herb that powers the nervous system in a centered, relaxed manner, always finding the middle way. It has a very solar effect, enhancing wellbeing, joy and openness, and letting go of traumatic experiences.

Oregano is a nerve tonic that calms, relaxes, removes tension, stress and anxiety and, most of all, balances and clears the nervous system. It is also antibacterial, antiviral, anti-parasitic and anti-fungal. As an antioxidant, it is extremely powerful, and as an antiviral, it can kill MRSA.

Lemon Balm is a great sedative and relaxant, completely reducing nervousness and being a great help in depression. It feeds the brain, eases pain, and keeps senility at bay in old age. It specifically calms down the sympathetic nervous system and cases of hyperadrenalism and hyperthyroidism, and has an affinity for the heart and stomach—high blood pressure, heart palpitations being some of the most severe examples of afflictions Lemon Balm can help with. Ultimately, any kind of nervousness can be addressed with Lemon Balm.

Sumach clears out stuck states of fear, panic, anxiety and desperation.

St. John's wort is a powerful herb for the nervous system, bringing luminous clarity and ease of presence, which many people find helpful in curing depression, anxiety and insomnia.

Motherwort is an emotional support herb that opens up our mental system to the raw nature of experience in a compassionate, emotionally stable manner.

Rhodiola Rosea is an adaptogen that improves mental endurance as well as the body's energy, and has been used to cure depression and improve long term moods.

Herbs for Headaches

Wood Betony is a brain restorative that works amazingly for tension headaches and migraines, and headaches of all sorts, easing tension, pain and anxiety.

Calamus relaxes and energizes the brain, and is great for all headaches and nerve issues.

Cayenne works directly with the central nervous system and stops pain, so it can cure headaches quickly, working especially well for cluster headaches.

Feverfew is a direct remedy for migraines and headaches, and has a calming, stress-reduction effect.

Allspice is a relaxing analgesic that calms the mind and body.

Borage is a stress tonic that helps the body deal with nervous tension, and is the perfect remedy for tension headaches.

Catnip is a very safe sedative that relaxes the body-mind and takes stress away.

Oregano is a nerve tonic that calms tension, nerves and anxiety, and works for headaches and migraines.

Black Cohosh is for dull, cold and aching headaches that are depression related.

Peony is for spasms and general sensory overstimulation, and for PMS.

Horseradish cures sinus headaches.

Lavender is good for stress-related headaches.

Lemon Balm cures anxiety and stress related headaches.

Lemon Verbena also calms nerves and anxiety.

Passionflower is a sedative, and thus calms anxiety and stress.

Rosemary is good for cluster headaches.

Sage is also good for cluster heaches, because, like Rosemary, it keeps the blood in proper circulation, and it also helps with hormonally related headaches and overeating headaches—in larger doses it's good for tension headaches.

Elder Flower is for hot and deep, tense headaches.

Rose Petal is for congested headaches that are hot and damn and come with a fever and bloating.

Licorice works well for all headaches, in many people, and is always good for headaches that result of tiredness and adrenal insufficiency.

Skullcap is a relaxing nervine and mild sedative that is great for very deep tension headaches, and anxiety and stress headaches.

Valerian is a good pain relief herb that is also a strong sedative that takes away anxiety and stress, and heals the nervous system, so it is a great headache cure.

Vervain is good for stress and tension headaches, takes pain away and has a healing effect on the nervous system, works well for PMS.

Yarrow is good for digestive headaches, dull and stagnant headaches, and headaches that are caused by aching teeth.

Mugwort works great for digestion headaches, with nausea and heaviness. Poplar works for hot headaches (it contains aspirin, so careful with allergic reactions and drug interactions).

White Willow Bark is another pain killing herb popular for headaches, also containing aspirin.

Ginger is great for cold headaches and virus related head pain, as well as headaches born of circulatory problems.

Clematis is for cluster headaches and good for migraines.

Dandelion is great for digestive headaches and for getting rid of stagnating heat.

Goldenrod is for stuffy allergy headaches and sinus infections.

Mullein takes pain away and is great for tension headaches, especially if neck and back tension is involved.

Oregon Grape Root is great for sinus infection headaches and liver congestion headaches.

Herbs for Digestion

Cinnamon is one of the most stabilizing herbs for the whole body-mind system, and it works for digestion as well. It balances and quickens digestion when needed, cures loss of appetite, indigestion and bloating.

Licorice evens everything out, balancing stomach acid and digestive juices.

Fennel seeds ease stomach cramps, nausea, flatulence, bloating and indigestion.

Turmeric keeps stomach processes balanced and lowers digestive inflammation.

Chamomile—prevents or relieves stomach cramps, calms the nervous system (including stress and anxiety), anti gas and bloating, helps nausea, heartburn and headaches.

Lemon balm helps with abdominal pain, bloating, and soothes the digestive and nervous systems.

Cardamon is a carminative (warming, and induces the expulsion of gas from the stomach and intestines), and a great healing herb for the stomach stomach and intestines, as well as inflammation and gas issues.

Caraway is also a carminative, warming, speeding up and improving digestion and reducing gas.

Also a carminative, Cumin improves digestion and reduces gas. Fennel, like the other carminatives, warms things and speeds up digestion while reducing gas.

Artichoke eases indigestion, bloating and gas, promotes bile flow, increases fat digestion and detoxifies the body.

Peppermint eases indigestion, relieves IBS, reduces spasms and pain.

Ginger strenghtens the body and cures indigestion, stimulates the stomach and increases the absorption of nutrients, absorbs toxins and helps the skin release them.

Mullein Leaf helps with a multitude of things: constipation, hemorrhoids, diarrhea and bladder infections.

Barberry Root is a bitter stomach tonic and a mild laxative.

Dill soothes indigestion and is a great digestion aid.

Lemon verbena improves digestion and gas problems, while easing stomach and intestine cramps.

Mashmallow and Psyllium seed balance bowel function, and soothe the gut. Flax seed is a balancing laxative.

Dandelion root and leaf improve digestion, stimulate digestion and are mild laxatives.

Yellow dock is a mild laxative and increases bile production.

Slippery Elm Bark is a mucilage that relieves IBS and soothes the rest of the digestive tract.

Activated Charcoal is great at absorbing toxins and poisons, and can get rid of many of the pathogens that cause food sickness. It bonds with any toxin or organism and carries it out of the body with the next bowel movement. Mix activated charcoal powder with water and drink, or use capsules.

Herbs for Colds

Astragalus is a good basis for fighting any cold or flu, being a strong, balanced adaptogen that supports the immune system in a variety of ways. The same could be said of any of the other supportive adaptogens.

Calamus also excels at removing colds, especially their source n the head, chest and throat, and directly fights infections while supporting the immune system.

Licorice is also an adaptogen, soothing, healing and supportive, and works as an expectorant and demulcent, relieving pain in mucus membranes.

Yarrow is a blood tonic that fights acute colds and flus and restores the body when severely attacked by cold symptoms—it is both cooling and warming, mastering fevers and body fluids.

Black Pepper is a strong, balancing herb that goes deep into any cold and fights it at the source, eliminating phlegm and weakness.

Turmeric is a balancing antiviral and antibacterial that goes to great lengths to support your body.

Ginger is a strong tonic that is powerfully anti-inflammatory and antioxidant, stops headaches, fly and cold symptoms, and returns the body to normal functioning through sweating and empowering the lymphatic system.

Cayenne is an incredibly heating herb that instantly lets you breathe better and reduces pain, gives energy, restarts the nervous system, the heart and the lymphatic system.

Cinnamon is a powerfully warming and balancing spice that fights colds, improves circulation and relieves congestion.

Cowslip also destroys phlegm and chest congestion.

Basil reduces fevers and helps alleviate the immediate symptoms of colds. Eucalyptus clears sinuses and respiratory infections.

Hyssop is another herb for clearing symptoms.

Horehound is the best herb for eliminating harsh mucus congestion of the airways. It also reduces headaches that stem from sinus infection.

Marjoram is another herb that clears congestion, as is horseradish.

Mullein improves breathing and eases sore throats.

Oregano tea revitalizes and stops coughing.

Spearmint clears coughs and bronchitis, Rosemary eases nose and chest congestion, Red Clover removes chest congestion and stops coughs, Thyme tea eases congestion and coughs, while Sage is effective for sore throats and coughs.

Echinacea is a classic flu and cold remedy, best taken at the onset of symptoms, but also effective throughout a cold, reducing its duration. Elderberry is another classic herb, an antiviral and anti-inflammatory.

Herbs for Fever

Yarrow reduces fever, increases perspiration and helps the body eliminate toxins—when put together in a tea with Peppermint, Ginger, Cayenne, Boneset and Elder flowers, you can powerfully handle bad fevers. Yarrow is the key to the rest of these herbs.

Ginger is a warming, stimulating herb that induces sweating and reduces very high fevers.

Boneset treats the worst of fevers, bone-shaking fevers and pain associated with the flu.

Black Elder eliminates toxins, lowers inflammation in the head and chest, lowers very high fevers and increases perspiration.

Peppermint tackles high fevers, and pacifies the mental aspect of being sick—reducing anxiety and bringing sleep and relaxation.

Catnip is another herb that soothes the mind, being a sedative traditionally used to cure fevers by increasing sweating. Combine with Mint and Sage for fevers that aren't too strong.

Feverfew is an anti-inflammatory that dilates blood vessels and relaxes your nervous system, making it a good choice for fevers that have a headache component.

Valerian is a mild sedative and gentle sleep aid.

White Willow is a classic fever remedy. Teas made from willow bark minimize high fevers and pain.

Echinacea is also a much appreciated herb that tackles strong infections and fevers, being an immune system stimulant with antiviral and antimicrobial powers.

Meadowsweet is a gentle fever herb that also reduces pain and digestive problems.

Herbs for Wounds and Cuts

Yarrow is the best open wound remedy. It is named after the legendary hero Achilles, and used to be carried into battle by warriors. It's great for deep wounds that bleed a lot, stopping the bleeding very quickly and uniting the edges of the wound. Yarrow also prevents inflammation, infection, and scarring. It is the single most important wound healing plant, with strong antiseptic functions that make it a great choice for animal bites and infections.

Calendula is an anti-inflammatory that keeps wounds clean, or cleans out old and infected wounds. It should be applied after bleeding has stopped.

Comfrey rebuilds tissues fast, but quite randomly. It does not help the edges of a wound find each other, the way Yarrow does, instead, it attempts to simply fill the wound with new tissue - often with quite surprisingly bad results. Comfrey is also likely to rebuild skin on the surface of a wound, while leaving infections to thrive underneath. There are uses for Comfrey, but not in the initial stages of healing.

Similarly, Goldenseal is good at sanitizing and sealing clean wounds, but when used on a dirty wound, it will seal all the dirt in. It can also seal an infection in—a very bad thing.

Plantain is a great wound cleaner, pulling any dirt out of the body and clearing infections, and also greatly regenerates tissue. White Pine is another herb with this ability.

Elecampane is an antiseptic and antibiotic that helps form a good scab, maintaining good aesthetics of the skin.

Turmeric reduces healing time and scarring, restores skin, and has even been used for cancer sores and diabetic ulcers. It is also anti-viral and anti-bacterial, and has been used against snakebites.

St. John's Wort should be used in wounds to areas that have lots of nerves, such as the eyes, ears, the fingers, toes, spine and genital area, as well as wounds that cause sharp pain. It protects nerves and, if you ever have a finger or limb surgically reattached, you should use St. John's Wort. It helps the nervous system know itself and piece itself back together.

Herbs for Head Injury

Yarrow should always be taken internally when there is head or spinal injury. It should also be religiously used after surgery to these areas, to prevent any kind of complications.

Calamus does wonders for mental presence and the subtle mental nerves that rule over mental processes and memory. It can bring everything back together following a head injury.

Black Cohosh helps the spine and neck come back online after injury, and it can also remove the mental darkness and clinging that comes with problems to the energy-transmitting structure, the neck and spine.

Wood Betony helps the brain recover, it is specifically useful for head injuries and concussions, or surgery. When there is lack of circulation in the brain, or lack of mental presence, Wood Betony also works very well.

Peony Root also restores thinking processes.

Goldenseal stops leakage from various internal wounds that can appear after brain injury, it seals them, and it does the same to spinal disks that have been torn or displaced.

Herbs for Broken Bones

Boneset is the great herb for setting broken bones and allowing the healing process to take place successfully.

True Solomon's Seal controls bone swelling and restores bone flexibility, remarkably aiding the recovery process in breaks. It restores the proper tension of ligaments, is great for healing the back, and the musculoskeletal system in general.

Comfrey is also known as Knitbone, and can set bones, but its wild regenerative powers can cause trouble, just as with wounds—leading to extra regeneration of non-bony tissues. It can be taken internally to power up the healing process.

Mullein lubricates the bones and eases their process of getting back into the right place, bringing them together.

Horsetail aids the healing of bones and cartilage.

Herbs for Burns and Sunburns

Plantain—pounded fresh leaves reduce pain and regenerate the skin.

Oats—make a poultice of oatmeat and water and use it to cover the area of the burn.

St John's Wort is antibacterial and antiviral, and has a long history of use for burns.

Sweet leaf is a hot herb that draws heat out of a burn. Chew the plant a bit, which releases its head, and apply it directly to the wound. Sweet leaf is particularly good in burns that produce cold sweat and shock.

Cabbage, crushed and mixed with a bit of oil, such as olive or coconut oil, and applied as a poultice, and changed often, nourishes and rebuilds the skin. The same can be done with Carrots and Apples.

Aloe is good for pain and inflammation and prevents infection.

Marhmallow makes a natural gel when boiled for ten minutes, and this covers and feeds the burn, reducing pain and inflammation.

Agrimony and Cinquefoil are for harsh burns that make you restrict your breathing. Applied directly, they heal the burn and the pain, allowing the nervous system to relax and resume the healing process.

Lavender has a long history of being used as a burn treatment—it's a disinfectant that quickens healing and reduces pain.

Nettle is an herb that burns the skin, but sometimes it takes a burning essence to treat a burn, and Nettle infusion or its fresh juice can be applied directly to burns. Nettle tea can also be used internally in the case of large, serious burns, which flood the bloodstream with damaged tissue protein. Nettle can help flush out these proteins and protects the kidneys—this is a serious matter, as people used to die from burns before dyalisis machines came along.

Herbs for Poisonous Bites

Plantain quickly pulls out venom and toxicity, and should be immediately applied to any kind of poisonous bite. Time is important with serious bites, and even apparently harmless stings could cause infection or an adverse reaction. Chew Plantain leaves and put them on the spot. It has been used for snake bites, and quickly heals insect bites.

Gentian treats anaphylactic shock, which is what you'd usually get from a bee sting, but can also occur due to certain foods—such as what someone allergic to peanuts may get in a worse case scenario. It empowers instincts and removes fear, exhaustion, and is a whole-body tonic, so being able to quickly take Gentian internally in case of anaphylactic shock can be a life-saver. For this purpose, Gentian tincture would have to be use, as a tea would take too long in case of shock.

St. John's Wort also has a long history of being used for poisonous bites, and should be added to poultices used for treatment whenever time allows it.

Herbs for Bruises, Strains and Sprains

Arnica is good for any kind of bruises, but works best for recent bruises, strains and sprains. It is specifically indicated for red and blue bruises with no broken skin, because when taken internally or placed on an open wound, it is toxic, causing irritation and excessive bleeding.

Yarrow is also for red and blue bruises, but should be used when the skin is also cut or perforated, or there is pooling of blood under the bruise.

Safflower is for deeper red and blue bruises, with a more infected, darker appearance. When the bruise is not recuperating, use Safflower.

For black and blue marks, tight or weak tendons, use True Solomon's Seal.

For a blue bruise, with swelling and edema, use Elder—especially for strains of the ankles and wrists.

Herbs for Boils and Abscesses

Plantain should always be used on abscesses, including tooth abscesses. Tooth pain is horrible, especially when there is an abscess, but Plantain easily takes care of it and draws out the infection.

Peach should be used on hot, dry boils. Make a strong tea by boiling two peach pits in a cup of water, simmering for ten minutes, and apply the tea as a compress and drink it for internal cleansing.

Slippery Elm bark, used as a poultice, was often used by Native Indians for boils, wounds, and skin disease. Make a paste with cold water, without boiling, and apply.

Thyme—heat up a strong thyme tea using a handful of thyme to half a liter of water. Apply a thyme compress to any abscess, boils, or swelling, and repeat when needed.

Elder pulls heat and its leaves can be used on boils, burns and abscesses.

Echinacea can be used externally, and internally as well, when the body seems to be habitually producing boils and abscesses.

Burdock has been used in Europe, India and China to treat abscesses. Pliny the Elder, the Roman naturalist, gives a formula that uses Plantain, Burdock, and Elder leaves for direct application on boils and abscesses.

Gravel Root tea can be used to take toxins out of the bloodstream, thereby removing an abscess. It is great at this.

Herbs for Tooth Health and Pain

Plantain can pull out infected and abscessed substances from the roots of teeth, healing a tooth directly where there would otherwise be a need for root canals.

Dandelion can restore and remineralize bones, even infected bones—which works for teeth, the alveolar bone, maxillae and the mandible.

White Oak Bark is a general tonic for dental health.

Self heal cures tooth decay when taken internally.

Gargle with Sage for chronic gum inflammation. Gargle with Echinacea for local healing.

Bloodroot has very powerful plaque fighting ability and removes the bacteria that rot teeth.

Herbs for Nerve Injuries

Chamomile is a great relaxant, it allows people to bear pain, so use a tea when injuries to nerve-rich areas occur.

As already mentioned, St. John's Wort is good for wounds to sensitive, nerve-rich spots, such as the eyes, ears, the fingers, toes, spine and genital area, as well as wounds that cause sharp pain.

Calamus can also be used for nerve pain, with strange, tingling sensations, and it is also an American Indian remedy for toothache.

Prickly Ash is for the most severe of pains, for unstoppable, agonizing pain. Prickly Ash Bark, chopped or powdered, and used as a poultice, applied directly to the affected area, is more effective than tea. It can also be used for toothache.

Wood Betony, taken internally, benefits the brain and nervous system, so it can help in nerve injuries.

Printed in Great Britain
by Amazon